GILLIAN GRAY

IRRITABLE BOWEL SYNDROME

The Ultimate Guide on How to Cure Irritable Bowel Syndrome, Learn All the Important Information about IBS and What You Can Do to Manage It

Descrierea CIP a Bibliotecii Naţionale a României
GILLIAN GRAY
　　IRRITABLE BOWEL SYNDROME. The Ultimate Guide on How to Cure Irritable Bowel Syndrome, Learn All the Important Information about IBS and What You Can Do to Manage It / Gillian Gray. – Bucharest: Editura My Ebook, 2020
　　ISBN

GILLIAN GRAY

IRRITABLE BOWEL SYNDROME

The Ultimate Guide on How to Cure Irritable Bowel Syndrome, Learn All the Important Information about IBS and What You Can Do to Manage It

My Ebook Publishing House
Bucharest, 2020

TABLE OF CONTENTS

INTRODUCTION

Everyone has an upset stomach from time to time.

You probably know the sort of thing I mean – sometimes you've got gas and at other times you feel queasy or nauseous. There may be times when you can't seem to go to the toilet for days, constipated as can be, but there are other days when diarrhea strikes and you can't stop going!

Although we all know that there are some foods or drinks that might prompt our digestive system to react in a certain way – a big meal of very spicy food sends many people scurrying to the bathroom for example – the only really predictable thing about our digestive system is its unpredictability.

However, because for most of us our digestive system acts the way we expect it to most of the time, we don't really give a great deal of thought to what our colon and gastrointestinal system is doing unless it is 'misbehaving'.

This is not the case for everyone however. A surprisingly high number – some reports suggest that it could be as many as one in five US citizens - suffers from a chronic condition called

Irritable Bowel Syndrome (IBS) and for these people, what their digestive system is doing can often dictate what they do too.

As with the majority of non-life threatening medical conditions, there are essentially two ways that you can deal with IBS.

Option one is to visit your doctor or other medical care professional, get a prescribed pharmaceutical medicine and take it. This option might be an effective way of managing your condition but as with many pharmaceutical situations and the drugs related to them, you have to consider the side effects before deciding whether this approach to IBS is the right one for you.

The second alternative is to do things the natural way, dealing with your condition using only treatment methods and substances that in many examples have been used for hundreds and thousands of years.

Hence, whilst I will highlight some medicines that your doctor is likely to prescribe for IBS and the possible adverse consequences of using them, the main focus of this book is very firmly fixed on giving you all the information you could ever need about dealing with IBS 100% naturally.

In doing this, the idea is to encourage you to at least try to handle irritable bowel syndrome naturally before turning to chemical-based pharmaceutical drugs because dealing with the problem naturally is simply a better way of doing so.

WHAT IS IRRITABLE BOWEL SYNDROME?

Irritable bowel syndrome is a chronic disorder (a long-term problem that could potentially last for life) that affects your gastrointestinal tract and intestines. It is a condition that is characterized by recurring problem in your stomach and bowels, often marked by regular bouts of diarrhea and/or constipation, stomach pain and spasms, bloating and gas etc.

In effect, people who suffer from IBS have intestines that either squeeze too hard or do not squeeze hard enough to eject waste materials from their body. Thus, there is a lack of the normal continual rhythm that characterizes the average human digestive system.

Research suggests that IBS sufferers appear to have a colon that is somehow more sensitive to a variety of different stimuli that have little or no effect on people who do not suffer from the condition. For example, certain foods that have no effect on other people can cause big problems for IBS sufferers.

Furthermore, stress is also known to be an extremely important contributory factor for many sufferers.

On top of this, there is some evidence that the immune system, the system body that fights infection and disease is also somehow involved in deciding who suffers from IBS and who does will not. It seems likely that the immune system also has a part to play in dictating how severe the condition is in any individual sufferer as well.

Irritable bowel syndrome is a condition that most commonly hits people between the years of 20 and 30, with women being twice as likely to suffer from the condition as their male counterparts.

One of the major difficulties attached to dealing with the problem is that whilst many the symptoms are easily recognizable, the actual cause of irritable bowels syndrome has not been fully established. For example, there are no signs of physical disease in the colon of most IBS sufferers, whilst there are no specific tests that can be used to diagnose the condition either.

Nevertheless, it is a fact that for many IBS sufferers, the symptoms do deteriorate after eating or when they are under stress, so this is a consideration which your doctor will take into account if they were attempting to diagnose whether you are suffering from irritable bowel syndrome or not.

In addition, irritable bowel syndrome is not really one recognizable medical condition at all as the term is used as a blanket to cover many different medicals symptoms that would usually be seen as nothing more than an upset stomach were they to occur in isolation.

What this means is that every imaginable symptom that you could possibly conceive of as a result of suffering an upset stomach is a symptom that you can associate with irritable bowel syndrome as well.

As suggested, IBS is a condition that can persist for many years, but the good news is, the disorder itself does not tend to get more serious or severe overtime. Whilst individual 'attacks' can vary in severity, the condition itself does not. Furthermore, under normal circumstances, IBS has nothing to do with and does not lead to more serious medical conditions such as cancer or inflammatory bowel disease.

It is a condition that has had several different monikers over the years, many of which are not normally used today.

Nevertheless, if you see reference to mucus colitis, nervous diarrhea, spastic colon or spastic colitis, you can be sure that the writer (it will almost certainly only be in written materials that you will see these terms nowadays) is referring to irritable bowel syndrome.

WHAT ARE THE MOST COMMON SYMPTOMS?

Initial diagnosis

As previously suggested, irritable bowel syndrome is not one recognizable illness, disease or infection. Instead, it is a collection of symptoms that are all grouped together under the same heading for the sake of convenience.

For this reason, there is a problem that when you have an upset stomach, this is almost always exactly what it is – nothing more or less than an upset stomach. And equally obviously, not everyone who suffers an upset stomach is a genuine irritable bowel syndrome sufferer.

For this reason, general descriptions of the symptoms attached to IBS are not always particularly helpful because a suggestion that a term such as 'changes in your bowel habits' is representative of IBS does not really get you much further forward.

Because most people who are suffering stomach or bowel problems need to know whether irritable bowel syndrome is their problem, it makes sense to analyze the symptoms in a little more depth.

In order to do so and in the interests of making the description of what IBS is as detailed as possible, I will highlight how your doctor might decide whether you're suffering from irritable bowel syndrome or not.

As suggested previously, there are no established tests which can be used to prove whether you are suffering from IBS or whether you have nothing more than an upset stomach. Consequently, the science or art of diagnosing irritable bowel syndrome is based upon discounting alternatives that produce IBS-like symptoms to eventually arrive at the correct conclusion. To do this, doctors use many different systems and criteria.

Whilst there are plenty of different algorithmic systems that doctors have used to diagnose IBS (including the Manning Criteria), many of these systems are now considered obsolete, having been replaced by the Rome III Criteria or process which was published in 2006.

This is therefore the system that we will use to try to formulate a reasonably accurate diagnostic symptom list for IBS.

As a patient, you would meet the basic criteria for IBS according to the Rome III process if your symptoms have persisted for a period of at least six months, assuming that during that period of time, you have suffered at least three bouts of difficulties or discomfort every month.

Furthermore, your doctor will be looking for a 'match' with at least two out of the three following statements:

• Your pain is relieved when you achieve a successful bowel movement;

• The pain you feel usually occurs at a time when you can identify consistency or appearance changes in your stools and

• Your pain also appears to be linked to alterations in the regularity with which you successfully achieve bowel movements as well.

With a match against two out of these three recognize symptoms of IBS established, your doctor would probably be satisfied that you appear to be suffering from IBS, but they would probe further to confirm the diagnosis.

This would be important because whilst these primary diagnostic requirements are important, they might suggest that irritable bowel syndrome is a condition of which regularity is a feature. This is however not necessarily true.

One of the characteristics of IBS that many sufferers find most frustrating or annoying is the fact that the condition is hardly ever regular. They never have the luxury of knowing what is going to happen next.

Hence, your doctor will probably probe a little deeper to establish whether the degree of irregularity that is characteristic of irritable bowel syndrome is present.

In order to do so, he or she would again look for two matches from this group, although even one match might sometimes be acceptable.

You probably have IBS if:

•Bowel movements often differ in consistency in size, sometimes being small, hard and bullet-like or perhaps thin, stringy or watery at other times;

•The physical action of passing a stool and the feelings associated with it differ from experience to experience. Sometimes, you may have to strain whilst at other times, the urge to go to the toilet hits you like a proverbial express train.

Furthermore, many IBS sufferers report that they often feel as if they have not passed the complete stool from their body as well;

•Bowel movements differ in frequency, sometimes happening two or three times every day (usually as diarrhea), whilst at other times, you may not need the bathroom more than once every three or four days;

•Many times, your stomach feels bloated or gas filled.

If any or more than one of these attendant symptoms are present, your doctor will probably diagnose irritable bowel syndrome.

However, this is still not the end of the story as there are various other symptoms that may or may not be indicative of IBS which your doctor might probe for.

For example, some people who have IBS suffer constipation that is immediately followed by diarrhea, accompanied by a degree of lower abdominal discomfort, whilst others might have the constipation and the pain but not diarrhea.

Then there are a wide range of 'symptoms' that your doctor may look for that are not necessarily symptoms of irritable bowel syndrome itself. Instead, many of these additional symptoms are in fact more like pointers to a possible cause of your condition instead of being a symptom of it.

For example, your doctor might question whether you have recently been under any excess stress or if you have been feeling anxious or depressed. If so, these are less likely to be symptoms of irritable bowel syndrome than causative factors.

However, the fact that something (in your doctors thinking, perhaps stress, fatigue or anxiety) has probably caused IBS is the genesis of a vicious circle. You are stressed so you developed IBS, and as a result of IBS, your stress has got even worse. After all, how can you feel relaxed and comfortable if you know that your digestive system can let you down without prior warning at any time and that you might need to find a toilet immediately when it does?

Your doctor might question whether you have suffered headaches or backache, sleeping problems or urinary difficulties. The latter might be relevant because especially when you have diarrhea, it is common that many people to need to urinate less often, hence this question.

Other folks suffer from sexual problems or heart irregularities and palpitations which at first glance would appear to have nothing to do with a gastrointestinal problem like irritable bowel syndrome.

However, as you will discover many times in this report, stress is generally considered to be an extremely important contributory factor for IBS. As sexual problems and heart palpitations are the kind of problems that healthcare professionals acknowledged to be indicative of stress, hence the question.

Testing for IBS

As previously suggested, irritable bowel syndrome is not a recognizable disease or illness nor is there a recognized test which can categorically establish whether someone is suffering from IBS or not.

Nevertheless, although 95% of the IBS diagnostic process will be based on the kind of questions highlighted in the previous section, there are a few tests that your doctor might carry out to rule out other conditions. In this way, whilst they cannot positively say with 100% certainty that you are suffering from irritable bowel syndrome, they can narrow it down to being a distinct possibility that you are.

The amount of testing that your doctor or hospital does depends on several factors, including your gender, age, your previous medical record, how severe your symptoms are, how often they appear, and so on.

For instance, I suggested that the most common IBS sufferer is likely to be a young woman in her 20s. Consequently, if the patient matches this age and gender profile, most doctors will do little more than a simple blood test to rule out the most likely alternatives before diagnosing irritable bowel syndrome.

If on the other hand the patient is a 60-year-old male, more detailed testing is likely to be needed as this individual is far less likely to have developed irritable bowel syndrome for the first time. The patient is the wrong gender and the wrong age, which tends to suggest that the condition is something other than IBS, hence more thorough testing would be called for.

Some of the tests that might be carried out to establish whether your problem is irritable bowel syndrome or not are full medical examinations and analyses of your complete medical history, detailed stool analysis and a complete or full blood count test.

And of course, depending upon the ailment or disease which your doctor suspects you may be suffering from, the range and number of tests that they conduct will vary from case to case.

Basically, with most or all of these tests, your doctor or medical specialist is trying to establish that irritable bowel syndrome is not your problem, usually based on the suspicion that something possibly far more serious is the cause of your current difficulties.

Remember, IBS is not a single recognizable disease and there is no specific test for it, so by definition, all of these tests must be for something else.

Questions to ask...

As is probably obvious by now, if your doctor runs a multitude of tests, it is because they suspect that your condition is not irritable bowel syndrome. Hence, there are questions that you should be prepared to ask your doctor when seeking their advice about what you suspect to be IBS.

For example, whether your doctor decides to carry out a multitude of tests or not, you need to establish whether your condition could be anything other than irritable bowel syndrome. Specifically, you need to ask about other, more serious conditions, especially colon cancer.

On the other hand, if your doctor does not ask you to undergo a program of testing and suggests that you are indeed suffering from irritable bowel syndrome, there are questions that you need to ask in this situation as well.

For instance, many patients who suffer from IBS will from time to time become constipated. In this situation, many people would be tempted to use an over-the-counter laxative to 'free up' their problem but you should not do so without asking your doctor whether this is okay.

As IBS is a condition that seems to be caused by over-sensitivity in your digestive system and colon, using laxatives may in fact make the condition worse, so don't consider using them before asking.

As you will read, one very effective way of dealing with irritable bowel syndrome is to change your diet (and your lifestyle) to one that is more amenable to your condition. It will do no harm to ask your doctor's advice about dietary matters because they will certainly have some ideas that might be useful to you.

HOW DOES WESTERN MEDICINE TREAT
IRRITABLE BOWEL SYNDROME?

Irritable bowel syndrome is not a condition that can be cured by standard medical practices, primarily because there is no single condition and there is therefore no single causative 'root' that can be attacked.

Instead, for anyone who suffers from IBS, it is all about managing their condition so that they can live a life that is as normal as possible.

Every individual irritable bowel syndrome sufferer is different. Thus, the factors that might cause one IBS sufferer to suffer diarrhea or constipation might have no effect whatsoever on others who have nevertheless been diagnosed with exactly the same condition.

For this reason, managing irritable bowel syndrome can involve one of many different changes or factors, with the changes or factors that are most appropriate to you depending upon the primary cause of your condition.

We will look at many of these potential changes later but before doing so, let us consider some of the medicinal solutions that your doctor might recommend to help you manage your irritable bowel syndrome problem.

Once again, the medicines that your doctor might prescribe or recommend will to a large extent depend upon the prevalence of symptoms that you as an individual display.

For example, if your primary problem is diarrhea, then the medicines that your doctor prescribes will target this particular aspect of your suffering. If on the other hand you suffer regular bouts of constipation, then prescribing a medicine to deal with diarrhea is going to be a very bad idea indeed! Obviously, your doctor would prescribe or recommend something more appropriate to your own personal situation and circumstances.

Of course, if you suspect irritable bowel syndrome and visit your doctor for a diagnosis (which is to be recommended), you already know what your primary symptoms are. After all, you have been living with them for several months, so who knows better than you?

Hence, from your own personal knowledge, you should be able to form some idea of the kind of medicines your doctor most needs to prescribe if you visit their office because you suspect that you have irritable bowel syndrome.

Medicines for diarrhea

If the primary symptom from which you suffer is diarrhea, your doctor is likely to prescribe one or a mixture of several different types of medicine.

The initial medicines to consider are anti-diarrheal pharmaceuticals such as Lomotil or Imodium.

The first of these brand-named products is a mixture of two chemicals, diphenoxylate and atropine. In combination, these two drugs slow intestinal movements, thereby interfering with the passage of matter through the digestive system as a method of reducing diarrhea.

In general terms, the worst side-effects that most people suffer after taking diphenoxylate are headaches, dizziness and drowsiness.

However, you should be aware that this particular substance is treated as a regulated narcotic drug in most Western countries, and that like all other narcotics, it can cause a feeling of being 'high' and euphoria with worsening drug dependency not being unknown either.

Furthermore, if you are taking a Monoamine oxidase inhibitor (an MOA) like phenelzine (Nardil) or procarbazine (Matulane), you should be aware that taken in combination, these drugs can cause severe high blood pressure which might in the worst case scenario lead to a stroke and/or death.

The active chemical ingredient in Imodium is Loperamide which works by putting the brakes on the muscular contractions in your intestine by limiting the activity of the opioid receptors in the muscles lining them.

As with most medicines, at normal dosage levels, Imodium is safe for 99.9% of people who take it. However, as it is a drug that is often available over the counter as well as by prescription, you do need to exercise a little more care if you are not under medical attention was taking this drug.

For example, if you start to take Imodium and your diarrhea persists for more than 24 hours, you should seek medical advice as the medicine is apparently not working.

In addition, Imodium can cause adverse side-effects such as dizziness, abdominal cramps or swelling, constipation, indigestion, nausea and vomiting and in a very small number of cases, total paralysis of the intestine. In all of these situations, you should seek immediate medical attention.

The next type of drug that your doctor might prescribe or recommend for getting rid of diarrhea is a bile binding agent such as cholestyramine. It is bile that stimulates the digestive actions of your colon so a drug of this nature that slows down the production of bile helps to prevent diarrhea.

The most common side-effect of taking this drug is perhaps the one that you might anticipate which is constipation. However, in less common cases, prolonged exposure might cause tooth discoloration and decay. Some people might suffer severe stomach pains, unexplained bleeding and have difficulty swallowing.

Furthermore, similarly prolonged exposure to the drug might increase the risk of suffering gallstones.

Medicines for constipation

As with diarrhea, there are several different types of medicines that might be prescribed or recommended by your doctor (remembering that many of these medicines are available over the counter, albeit in slightly weaker forms than your doctor will subscribe).

The most common medicines are:

Lubiprostone is a drug that works by increasing the amount of fluid in your digestive system, thereby making your stools softer which in turn makes it easier for bowel movements to occur. The most common side effects of this drug are nausea and diarrhea, although decreased appetite and rashes can sometimes result from taking Lubiprostone too.

In addition, various different types of laxatives may be prescribed or recommended, including:

• Over-the-counter osmotic laxatives (Milk of Magnesia etc) which add additional fluids to stools to make them softer and easier to pass;

• Stimulant laxatives (Senokot and Correctol) that speed your digestive system up and

• Polyethylene glycol which enables stools to retain more fluid.

With all of these medicines, the major potential side effect is diarrhea, although long-term use of laxatives can lead to other potentially more serious side effects such as dehydration, electrolyte imbalance and in more extreme examples, laxative dependence, a situation where you can never go to the toilet without using laxatives first (or perhaps become genuinely addicted to them).

For cramping and pain

If a symptom of your irritable bowel syndrome is constant pain or stomach cramps, your doctor may prescribe or recommend anticholinergics or antispasmodic drugs such as dicyclomine. Drugs of this nature have a wide range of potential adverse side-effects, including flushing of the face, headache, dry mouth, sleeping difficulties, constipation, increased sensitivity to light and a constant thirst together with decreased sweating.

In addition, perhaps the best-known antispasmodic drug Bentyl has other potential side-effects such as dry eyes and stomach ache. For this reason, if you have a previous history of serious eye problems such as glaucoma, you need to make sure that your doctor is aware of these problems as the medicine may react with other drugs or exacerbate your problem.

Drugs for mental difficulties

As suggested earlier in the report, it is generally agreed that one of the primary causative factors involved in irritable bowel syndrome is stress or anxiety. Consequently, if this is considered to be a major cause of your IBS problems, your doctor may be tempted to prescribe drugs to help you get over the problem with the most likely candidate being antidepressants.

Leaving aside for the moment the fact that stress and anxiety are *not* the same as depression (which is a clinical condition) and are not therefore necessarily treatable with drugs designed to alleviate depression, many of the best-known antidepressant drugs have a very long list of potential adverse side-effects attached to them.

For example, the majority of antidepressant drugs that are prescribed nowadays are 'Selective serotonin reuptake inhibitors' (SSRIs) with perhaps the best-known of these being Prozac. The most common side- effects of drugs like Prozac are nausea, agitation and headaches, but other more serious side-effects are relatively common as well.

For example, sexual problems such as loss of libido, inability to achieve orgasm and erectile dysfunction are all relatively common, whilst all SSRIs have been associated with weight gain in both male and female patients.

On top of all of this, there is increasing evidence that people are becoming ever more dependent upon drugs like

Prozac, evidence which many people suggest is supported by the fact that in 2005, antidepressants became the most widely prescribed drug in the USA.

Although some doctors welcome this as a sign that people were more willing to seek help and assistance than previously, the majority view this as a sign of increasing dependence on antidepressants as a daily 'crutch', something that is becoming an ever more 'normal' aspect of society.

In short, if there is a stress element involved in your irritable bowel syndrome problem there is a valid to suggest that the last thing you should be doing is seeking a solution provided by antidepressants. The chances of these drugs bringing you any significant long-term benefits are probably very slim whilst there is a significant degree of doubt as to the efficacy of prescribing antidepressants for stress or anxiety in the first place.

The bottom line is...

There are many different drugs that your doctor might prescribe or recommend if he or she decides that you have irritable bowel syndrome. However, all of these drugs will manage your condition in one way or another rather than 'curing' it and there are many other ways of managing your condition that do not involve potentially harmful drugs.

Which of course brings us to the second major consideration to be borne in mind. All of the drugs highlighted in this section of the report do have potential side-effects ranging from the unpleasant to the positively dangerous.

In addition, because medicating yourself to manage your condition is such a fine balancing act, there will be times that the medicine you are taking will cause as many problems as it solves. For example, there may be times when constipation forces you to take a laxative, in which case you end up with diarrhea an hour or two later (if t takes that long!), so you have gone from one extreme to the other.

This is surely not a situation that you want to find yourself in because one miserable situation is not a great deal better than the other.

This is one major reason why looking at irritable bowel syndrome on the 'big picture' basis and dealing with it as a condition that tells you that you need to change your lifestyle is a far more sensible approach than medicating yourself.

By making appropriate lifestyle changes instead of turning to pharmaceutical drugs, you attack the problem at the root cause, rather than simply dealing with the symptoms.

Although there is no real 'cure' for IBS, the fact is that if you change as many of the factors that cause your condition as you can, you reduce the likelihood and frequency of irritable bowel syndrome causing difficulties in the future.

APPROACHING IRRITABLE BOWEL SYNDROME A BIT MORE THAN HOLISTICALLY...

Adopting a holistic approach to any medical condition or ailment suggests trying to deal with that condition on a 'whole-body' basis.

However, in this particular example, I would extend this from dealing only with matters that are concerned with your body to considering appropriate factors drawn from every aspect of your life too.

As a very simple example, we have already mentioned on many occasions that stress is generally believed to be one of the major causes of irritable bowel syndrome. Hence, if you can take actions that reduce the level of stress that you feel on a daily basis, you immediately remove one main factor that is causing your problem from the picture.

Somewhat obviously, diet is also another major consideration because any medical condition that is focused on your ability to pass food and waste materials through your digestive system without problems must be affected by your diet.

Hence, dealing with irritable bowel syndrome naturally is more to do with identifying the causes of your condition and then doing something about changing those causes for the better instead of only focusing on offsetting the worst effects of your condition.

CONTROLLING IRRITABLE BOWEL SYNDROME THROUGH DIET

If you are an irritable bowel syndrome sufferer, it is instinctively obvious that your diet plays a major factor in deciding how well or how sick you feel on any given day.

Consequently, it is likely that you have already searched for appropriate dietary information, details of the foods that you can and cannot eat that can help you to reduce the number of attacks you suffer as an irritable bowel syndrome sufferer. If so, I would wager that you have been somewhat disappointed with most of the information you have found because from my own research, I have found most of the information available to be vague, generalized and often little more than a wild stab in the dark at what might or might not work.

For example, you may have seen general advice that a high fiber diet or a diet that is rich in vegetables is good for someone who suffers from IBS. Whilst this might be true for a small percentage of sufferers, it is likely to be very small percentage indeed. A high fiber diet is the last thing you need if your condition is one where diarrhea or both diarrhea and constipation are present. Furthermore, if eating vegetables is a good idea, what kind of vegetables should they be?

One of the problems seems to be that the majority of IBS sufferers know that there are certain foods which irritate them and certain foods that they can eat almost every day without any problems whatsoever. However, in between these two categories, there are many foodstuffs that irritable bowel syndrome patients can eat one day, but not the next.

This leads to a good degree of confusion and a certain lack of clarity because there seems to be no logic in a scenario where you can eat something one day but not the next. Hence, some sufferers spend many fruitless hours trying to come up with a list of specific foods that cause them problems, whereas a lot of the time, compiling a list of this nature is almost impossible.

Allied to this is the fact that because irritable bowel syndrome is not one recognizable disease or condition, every individual sufferer is different. It might therefore be valid to ask, is there such a thing as a *generalized* IBS diet that will help at least the majority of sufferers, if not all of them?

Fortunately, the answer to the question is affirmative because although IBS is an individualized condition, it is not so individualized that some general dietary strategy that will work for most IBS sufferers cannot be formulated.

The first thing to understand is that you should try to get away from the idea of one single item of food (or drink) being your irritable bowel syndrome trigger. Instead of thinking of single, particular items of food as being triggers you should instead try to think in terms of food or drink groups.

Every different food or beverage group is either a gastrointestinal irritant or stimulant and each group will therefore be one that you should be including in your diet regularly or rarely, depending upon your own condition.

If you classify foods and beverages in groups in this way, it enables you to create a diet plan that does not focus on a very small, limited number of foods that you know to be (at least relatively) safe as far as your IBS is concerned.

On the other hand, it does allow you to eat a balanced, healthy diet, one that provides the variety and interest levels that you need in order to ensure that living with IBS does not get you down too much.

Remember what we have already said about anxiety and stress? If every day is miserable because you can never eat the kind of foods that you want to eat, this will inevitably increase your stress or anxiety levels. This further exacerbates your problem, thus it is clear that being able to eat a balanced but varied diet is extremely important both psychologically and physically.

In a nutshell, the best kind of diet for the majority of irritable bowel syndrome sufferers is one that is high in soluble fiber and low fat foods that are not likely to trigger an adverse gastrointestinal reaction. On the other hand, foods that are featured in the 'triggers' group should only ever be eaten rarely, if at all.

Soluble fiber foods

Most people are aware of the concept of food containing fiber, but what you might not be so clear is the fact that there are different types of food fiber. On the one hand, you have the kind of food fiber with which most people are familiar, the kind of fiber that you introduce to your diet by eating bran, whole grains and raw vegetables.

However, whilst for the majority of people, this is exactly the kind of fiber that they need (as most people eat far too little) it is the last thing that you need. Insoluble fiber or roughage of this type stimulates your digestive system pretty strongly, which is not good if you suffer from IBS.

What you need is soluble fiber as this form of fiber is still remarkably good for you with the ability to provide all of the vitamins and nutrients you need, but at the same time, it does not naturally irritate or stimulate your gastrointestinal tract.

What you are looking at here is a food group that contains foods such as rice, pasta, noodles, barley, soy, cornmeal, potatoes, yams, carrots, sweet potatoes, mushrooms, chestnuts and avocados. You will probably understand that these are all foods that are most commonly considered to be starchy foods, which is exactly what we are talking about when discussing soluble fiber foods.

Make foods of this type the main cornerstone of your irritable bowel syndrome diet and you have already taken a significant step towards reducing the severity of your symptoms and the regularity of attacks.

These foods are soluble because they have the ability to absorb excess liquids whilst passing through your colon, meaning that whilst they prevent diarrhea, they also gently stretch the muscles of your digestive tract as they pass through (gentle because the fluid makes these materials soft).

Consequently, eating foods of this nature promotes normal digestion. Hence, even if the prevalent symptom of your IBS is constipation, the fact that the fecal matter passing through your gastrointestinal tract is a soft and malleable 'gel' (rather than the normal 'bullets' or 'bricks') means that a diet rich in soluble fiber foods should reduce your problems as well.

The other major plus point of soluble fiber foods is the fact that eating foods of this nature brings regularity to your system, so you do not suffer the stomach cramps and pains that you might otherwise suffer. A diet that is rich in soluble fiber ensures that the consistency of the matter passing through your system always remains reasonably stable. Consequently, the pain that you might previously have become so used to should become a thing of the past relatively quickly.

As a general rule, you should always eat your soluble fiber first at any meal and if you need to snack between meals, try to snack on soluble fiber foods as well.

Insoluble fiber foods are necessary too, but...

In addition to soluble fiber foods, you do of course need to take on board some foods that contain insoluble fiber as well. After all, it would not be a very healthy diet that cut out fruit and vegetables entirely nor would it be a very interesting way of living your life either.

However, the keynote here is moderation. Whenever you are eating foods that are high in insoluble fiber (which are any foodstuffs that are stated to be high or even moderately high in fiber, because that almost always means roughage), you should do so in small portions and take your time when you're eating.

By eating small and slowly, you do not overload your system with too much of any one particular high-fiber foodstuff or a combination of them that might come back to bite you an hour or two later!

As an example, most vegetables (greens, peas, beans, corn, cabbage, broccoli, cauliflower etc) are insoluble fiber rich and you should therefore only eat a small portion of vegetables with a large portion of soluble fiber foodstuffs, rather than the other way round. The same rule applies to fresh fruit such as oranges, grapefruit, cherries, melons and pineapples. Once again, all of these fruits are rich in insoluble fiber, so take it easy.

Incidentally, if you do want to eat fruit, apples, peaches, apricots and pears are all far safer if you eat them after removing the skin, because with these fruits, most of the fiber is in the peel.

The 'go there at your peril' or triggers list...

The third list of foods are those that you really should avoid because these are all trigger foods that cause most people who suffer IBS problems to a greater or lesser extent.

In this category, you would include red meat, dairy products (even low- fat yoghurt is likely to irritate your stomach), egg yolks, French fries, onion rings, croissants, pastries, biscuits and so on. In effect, anything that is high in unsaturated fats should be a no-no or at least make sure that you eat high-fat foodstuffs only very, very occasionally and that if you do so, you are prepared for some kind of adverse reaction.

Avoid coffee (caffeine causes your stomach to contract, but even decaffeinated coffee should be avoided), alcohol, carbonated drinks and artificial sweeteners as well.

All of these contain chemicals or enzymes that are well-known stomach irritants, the kind of substances that are likely to cause anyone who suffers from irritable bowel syndrome a very unpleasant reaction.

Monosodium glutamate is also likely to cause irritation or stimulation of the gastrointestinal tract for almost any IBS sufferer, so be wary of eating fast food or processed foods that might contain MSG.

Final dietary thoughts...

It's a fact that no one wants to spend the rest of their life eating nothing but rice and pasta. It is also true that you have to include other foods in your diet in order to ensure that you take on board the necessary vitamins, minerals and nutrients that you need to maintain general good health and to have enough energy to enjoy your life.

Nevertheless, beyond soluble fiber foods, you have to learn to eat in moderation. You should also keep an eye on what you are eating on a daily basis (perhaps keeping a food diary might help) so that you can keep a record of any foodstuffs which have caused an adverse reaction.

In this way, you can reduce the amount of that particular food that you eat next time (you may simply have overindulged) or remove it from your future eating plans entirely.

One final tip is to start reading the labels of every food that you buy at your local supermarket or store because many of these foods will contain additives and preservatives, whilst some might contain vegetable or meat matter that the manufacture conveniently forgot to mention on the front of the can!

STRESS MANAGEMENT IS CRITICAL

When you are stressed or anxious, your body naturally produces excessive amounts of adrenalin which is a natural hormone that the body secretes in response to any increased emotional reaction such as excitement or anxiety.

For an irritable bowel syndrome sufferer, having an excess of adrenalin flowing round your body is a very bad idea because adrenalin has the capability of stimulating or upsetting the contractions of your stomach very quickly.

As a natural symptom of irritable bowel syndrome is to suffer irregular contractions of the gastrointestinal tract anyway, anything that stimulates further irregularity or unexpected increases in contractions is by definition bad. Thus, it should be easier to understand why stress is such a problem for people who suffer from IBS and why you need to bring it under control as quickly and as effectively as possible.

Why you must get a good night's sleep...

Whether you suffer from IBS or not, it is a fact that most people are not at their best if they have not had enough sleep. People who are tired tend to be far more irritable with correspondingly low stress-tolerance levels, whilst general fatigue often has a habit of turning smaller problems into larger ones that cause further anxiety and upset.

In terms of IBS, the importance of a good night's sleep has been proven by research that indicates a clear correlation between the incidence of early morning IBS attacks and poor sleep. In fact, the relationship was established to such an extent that a very clear pattern of association between poor sleep and raised incidences of IBS attacks is accepted as fact.

Specifically, most of these studies indicate that anyone who suffers from irritable bowel syndrome that manages to get more than eight hours sleep a night does not suffer increased stress and concomitant attack levels the next day, whereas people who sleep for less than eight hours a night do.

The message from this could not be clearer. You must ensure that you have at least eight hours restful sleep every night if you want to maximize your chances of minimizing stress, thereby reducing the chances of IBS attacks.

Yoga, meditation and deep breathing...

There are many practices like yoga and meditation that focus on training you how to get the best out of yourself and an integral part of most of these practices is acquiring the ability to relax deeply and thoroughly.

Hence, it is a fact that if you take up yoga or meditation, you are likely to learn many skills that will help you to relax and also overcome stressful situations far more effectively than you might otherwise do.

The best part about learning a form such as yoga or meditation is that whereas a few years ago, the only way of doing so would have been to learn from a book or to join a local class, there are nowadays many other options available with a plethora of information available for free on the internet.

The advantage of this is that you can pick up everything you need to know to start learning the basics of either yoga or meditation at home and in your own time. Based on your experiences during this acclimatization period, you can decide whether to take it further by seeking a local class or group where you can take your studies to the next level in a controlled and disciplined environment.

By following this initial study pattern, you ensure that you get the most out of whatever you are doing. This is very important as you have a very specific objective in learning either yoga or meditation, which is to relax, and this could be far easier if you are confident and enjoying herself.

As a starting point, I would suggest that you take some time to study the information about yoga on this website as all of the basics that you need are here.

Alternatively, some people prefer the slightly more sedentary approach to learning relaxation and mental discipline adopted by meditation over the more exercise based approach of yoga.

If this is the case, the same proviso applies once again. All of the information that you need to get started can be found on the net, with this being a very good place to start.

Both yoga and meditation put great emphasis on the importance of learning how to breathe properly can help you to master the art of relaxation.

Moreover, having the knowledge and the ability to breathe deeply and slowly at those times when stress seems imminent is an invaluable gift. There no doubt that for the
48

majority of people, the ability to stand back from such a situation in an effort to regain control before stress hits is a difficult one to master. However, if you can do so, it is one most effective ways of making sure that it never does.

In my own efforts to master the art of effective deep breathing, I found this website to be particularly valuable because it teaches a method of deep breathing that becomes almost involuntary that makes the whole thing easier. I would however also recommend that you should look at this page as well because there is also plenty of invaluable information here too.

Whether you ultimately decide that yoga or meditation is more 'your thing' than the alternative, the crucial thing to remember is to focus on learning as much as you can about mastering your emotions so that you can relax on demand. If you can do this effectively, you have acquired the ability to walk away from 95% of situations or scenarios that might have caused distress and anxiety in the past.

In this case, you have taken another giant (and completely natural) step towards bringing your irritable bowel syndrome under control by removing yet another everyday situation that might otherwise spark an IBS attack.

You may not be able to cure IBS, but if you can remove most of the factors that cause it from your life, it's the next best thing.

Hypnotherapy for overcoming IBS...

Most people have a pretty jaundiced view of what hypnosis is and what it does, probably colored by the fact that the sum total of their exposure to hypnosis has done little to convince them of its very real benefits.

They have probably spent time watching a stage hypnosis show where people did seemingly absurd or crazy things, or perhaps their ideas came from some old black-and-white movie peopled by a hypnotist armed with a swinging fob watch, a top hat and a ludicrous moustache!

For people who have no real experience of hypnosis, it might therefore come as a surprise to know that hypnosis as a form of a valid medical treatment has been approved by the American Medical Association for just over 50 years!

However, hypnosis was not invented 50 years ago, or even a couple of centuries ago. Hypnosis as a treatment form for both medical and psychiatric problems is one that has been used across thousands of years of history, although in more recent times, the 'father' of modern hypnotism is generally agreed to be Mesmer who came up with the method of hypnotism that is still recognizable today.

What hypnotism attempts to do is get past the conscious mind with which we make every day decisions to communicate with the subconscious mind from where, in fact, the vast majority of your life is controlled.

To get some idea of the difference between the conscious and subconscious, imagine that you are going to drive the kids to school in the morning.

You make a conscious decision to get out of bed, to make the breakfast and to get the car out of the garage. However, as soon as you start to drive, you no longer have to think of the actions that you have to undertake in order to make the car move from your home to the school.

The action of turning the steering wheel, using the gearshift and operating the brakes are all skills that you learned before consigning them to your subconscious mind when you no longer needed to think about them on a conscious level.

Every human being does this with dozens of learned experiences every day, so that most people have a subconscious mind that is packed with actions that control almost everything they do (without thinking) on a daily basis.

However, whilst hypnosis (or hypnotherapy as it is more correctly called when it is used as a form of treatment) is generally thought to be related to the mind only, it is a fact that the body of every human being is controlled by their mind. Your subconscious mind is driving the car, but your hands are operating the steering wheel and the gear shift, so the relationship between your mind and your body cannot be ignored or denied.

Another common mistake that people make when they consider hypnosis is to think that people who are hypnotized unconscious or asleep. Nothing could be further than truth because people in a hypnotized state are super-conscious, extremely highly attuned to every word and suggestion the hypnotist or hypnotherapist makes.

However, in this hypnotized stake (and it is suggested that 90% of us can be hypnotized), most people report being far more in-tune with their body and their internal feelings, emotions and desires as the outside world is effectively shut out. Consequently, hypnotherapy is extremely effective as a way of educating and communicating with patients at a subconscious level, teaching them how to relax when faced with a stressful situation without thinking.

But the power of hypnotherapy or hypnosis goes much further than this, because whilst you are in a trance, you are infinitely more suggestible than you will ever be whilst you are awake. In a suggestible state like this, you are far more open to an acceptance of new ideas and thoughts, ideas that you might immediately reject on a conscious level.

Hence, once you are in this suggestible stake, a good hypnotherapist will be able to convince you that your IBS problem is not really such a big problem at all, and that through the power of positive thinking and actions, you can control and ultimately defeat it.

If you were fully conscious, you would probably reject this idea out of hand. However, under hypnosis, you will not only accept it but also embrace and 'stash it away' deep in your sub-conscious as a guiding principle for the future.

In effect, in the same way that you just accept driving a car is something that you can do without giving it a second thought, hypnosis allows you to adopt a very similar attitude and approach to irritable bowel syndrome.

In future, your subconscious will 'tell' you that it is something you can manage by yourself, something that you can eventually defeat and you will probably never entertain a dissenting thought about either of these beliefs.

In short, hypnosis or hypnotherapy is one of the most powerful strategies for learning how to handle and deal with stress and for training your subconscious to deal with IBS in a totally 'can-do' matter- of-fact way at the same time.

In order to learn more about hypnosis or hypnotherapy, the best option is to find a professionally qualified hypnotherapist in your own town or city by using Google maps. As an example and as an indication that it is not only the major cities where you will find hypnotherapists, these are the results of a Google search for 'portland hypnotherapists':

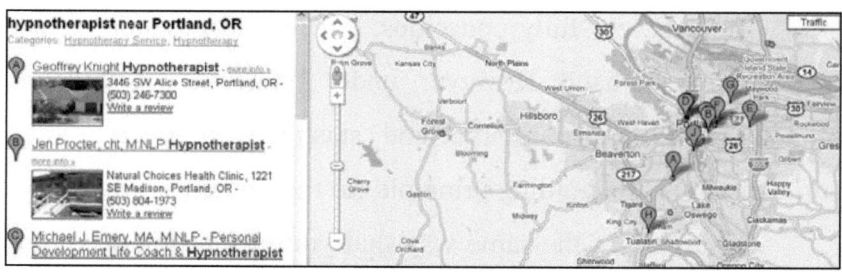

To back up these suggestions, there is now strong scientific evidence that hypnotherapy has a direct benefit for people who are suffering from irritable bowel syndrome too. The latest evidence can be seen by following the links here and

<u>here</u> but these are just the latest results following 15 years of solid research and study in many different countries.

In fact, the connection between controlling irritable bowel syndrome and hypnosis is now so strong that it has been suggested (by <u>Adriane</u> <u>Fugh-Berman, MD</u>) that hypnotherapy should be the first alternative treatment of choice after traditional Western medicine has failed.

Hypnotherapy might just be the most effective way of dealing with irritable bowel syndrome. If your problem is really getting you down, it is selling something that I would recommend you should try at least once.

I can't emphasize enough…

It seems likely that stress and anxiety is the number one cause of irritable bowel syndrome in 90% of sufferers.

Whilst poor dietary choices will not help, the theory that stress is the dominant factor that causes the condition is given credence by the fact that many IBS sufferers find that there are foods they can eat perfectly normally when they are calm and relaxed. However, exactly the same foods will cause a major adverse reaction when they are stressed and under pressure, so the only possible conclusion to draw is that stress is the deciding factor in dictating their reaction.

All the strategies that you have read of in the chapter will help to reduce the amount of stress that you feel in your life because you have to accept that you cannot remove every potentially stressful situation from your day-to-day existence. Instead, you have to learn to deal with stress and to conquer it.

Adopt the techniques and ideas that you have read of in this chapter, and getting on top of stress, becoming a master of it, should become progressively easier.

WHAT DOES TRADITIONAL CHINESE MEDICINE TELL US ABOUT IBS?

The answer to this question is… Nothing!

Despite medical expertise that goes back many thousands years more than the accumulated medical knowledge that we have acquired in the West, traditional Chinese medicine has nothing to say about irritable bowel syndrome at all!

However, on further investigation, the reason becomes clear.

As suggested many times in this report, there is no such illness or disease as irritable bowel syndrome as the phrase itself is a blanket, 'catch-all' term that covers a wide range of symptoms as opposed to one specific condition.

Thus, traditional Eastern medicine adopts a completely different approach to dealing with IBS than would a Western doctor. Instead of trying to pull every symptom of IBS together under the same heading, Eastern medicine works by isolating and then treating each individual symptom separately.

In this way, every individual IBS sufferer is treated for exactly the symptoms that they personally exhibit, rather than being treated as just another person who has a medical condition of some sort.

This approach makes far more sense than does the approach of the Western medical establishment who medicate patients that suffer from IBS as if it is a single, recognizable condition.

However, traditional Chinese medicine will approach your problem in two slightly different directions.

Firstly, a qualified practitioner of Chinese medicine would isolate each individual symptom that you suffer from.

Secondly, because traditional Oriental medicine works on the basis of triggering your own healing mechanisms rather than introducing outside substances in an attempt to heal you, your practitioner will look for the source of the weaknesses that are causing those symptoms, because that is where treatment is needed.

Armed with this information, he or she can then design a suitable program of treatment for you.

For example, you might believe that constipation is constipation.

Chinese medicine would not agree with you however, because according to traditional Chinese beliefs, the root cause of constipation falls into one of two categories, either excess type constipation or deficiency type.

The first job would therefore be to decide what kind of constipation you have. Once your therapist has isolated which specific type of constipation you are suffering from, then and only then will they decide upon the most appropriate form of treatment.

To continue with the same example, there are two subcategories of excess type constipation, both of which are reported to respond very well to acupuncture. However, whilst acupuncture will still work for deficiency type constipation, the benefits will be slow to develop and it is more likely that your therapist will recommend different types of herbal remedies as opposed to acupuncture for deficiency type constipation.

From this simple example, you can begin to see how the approach of traditional Chinese medicine is radically different to that of the medical profession in the West.

Whilst this form of treatment is aimed at managing your condition rather than curing it, this is probably the only real similarity between the two methods of dealing with IBS.

Of course, the most important question is, how effective is Chinese medicine in treating irritable bowel syndrome?

The answer is, most sufferers report extremely good results from various different forms of traditional treatment such as acupuncture, Chinese herbal remedies and in some cases, a little-known practice called moxibustion (the burning of mugwort on appropriate acupuncture points of the body), although this latter treatment is used very rarely.

Whilst there are no doubt some people who are still suspicious or a little nervous of considering using alternative forms of treatment like traditional Chinese medicine, there is plenty of evidence that using acupuncture or acupressure can help deal with a wide range of medical conditions (including IBS) in a completely natural and non-invasive way.

Once again, if you want to find a suitable Chinese therapist or acupuncturist, use Google maps or the Yellow Pages to find someone in your neighborhood. All of these treatments and non-invasive, so you have nothing to lose by trying.

SUPPLEMENTS AND HERBS FOR IBS

Supplements

There are quite a few supplements that you can use to help manage your condition, with some of them focusing on things that we have already dealt with, whilst others are more herbal in nature. I will therefore highlight the latter in the next section.

However, you already know that including soluble fiber in your diet is essential. Some people choose to do this by using supplements to top up the amount of soluble fiber they ingest in the food that they eat. One recommended supplement to consider is Ready Fiber whilst there is a list of several more supplements of this nature here.

Another supplemental source that is often effective for dealing with IBS are Probiotics such as acidophilus. These are cultures that help to control the growth of gastrointestinal flora which in turn helps to regulate the behavior of your stomach, helping to prevent the worst effects of irritable bowel syndrome developing.

Probiotics work particularly well when teamed with Prebiotics as the latter encourage the growth of the former (hence *pre*biotics), so if possible, you should therefore try to use the two in combination for best results.

Digestive enzymes like Beano can be very helpful when taken with a meal, especially if that meal contains more fat then you are used to eating or an excess of insoluble fiber foods. Digestive enzymes of this type help your body to break down the sugars present in your food, which prevents these sugars being deposited in your stomach undigested. If this happens, it presents the sugar with the opportunity of fermenting, thus producing gas, discomfort and other unpleasant side-effects.

Many IBS sufferers are deficient in trace minerals, particularly magnesium and calcium. However, because these two trace elements are counteractive of one another, it is important to know which you are deficient in before taking mineral supplements.

For instance, whilst calcium has a constipating effect, magnesium acts as a laxative. As long as you have a suitable balance between the two, your gastrointestinal tract will also remain in balance. If however one predominates over the other, then you have an obvious problem.

Herbs for irritable bowel syndrome

Peppermint oil is commonly used as a treatment for IBS as it is believed to reduce the bloating and abdominal pain often associated with the condition. This is believed to be connected to the fact that modern Peppermint contains a high concentration of menthol and methyl salicylate which both have noted antispasmodic qualities.

Peppermint oil is available in many different formats but if you plan to take this particular herbal supplement, be sure that you only do so in the form of enteric coated capsules. These capsules will stay intact until they arrive at their intended destination within your body, whereas using peppermint oil in any other form risks indigestion and heartburn (which is really not going to help anyone who suffers IBS).

Ginger is a herbal remedy that has been used for thousands of years and over those years, Ginger has established itself as a very effective substance for dealing with a wide range of digestive and gastrointestinal problems. For example, studies have indicated that Ginger is very capable of reducing the nausea associated with morning sickness or the after-effects of chemo or radiotherapy.

Caraway has been used for hundreds (perhaps even thousands) of years as a treatment for indigestion, colic and some nervous disorders.

Furthermore, caraway has anti-spasmodic and anti-microbial characteristics that enable it to help calm your stomach whilst also stimulating the proper production of gastric juices. It is also believed that chemicals in caraway seeds can help to soothe your gastric tract whilst helping to get rid of excess gas too.

Chamomile has anti-bacterial, anti-fungal, anti-inflammatory and anti- spasmodic characteristics, as well as being a natural sedative. Most commonly, the majority of people drink extract of chamomile as a tea, with plenty of research in recent years adding additional evidence for the calming and soothing effects of chamomile.

Fennel was used as a herbal remedy thousands of years ago in ancient China, with plenty of European evidence as to its efficacy as well. Once again, fennel is known to possess strong anti-spasmodic qualities.

In addition, the volatile oils in fennel make it extremely beneficial for anyone suffering from gastrointestinal problems, bowel irregularities (studies have indicated that it helps to control contractions in the small intestine), colic, heartburn and indigestion.

Fennel is one of the strongest herbs for reducing gas and bloating, which represent a couple of the more upsetting or uncomfortable characteristics of suffering from IBS. Furthermore, as you can drink fennel as a tea as well – it has a very pleasant mild licorice taste – it is another herbal remedy that it is easy to live with and use.

Oregano contains two volatile oils that are known anti-spasmodics. Including oregano in your diet will therefore help to reduce the painful stomach cramps that are commonly associated with suffering an IBS attack.

Anise has been used as an aid to digestion since the time of the ancient Greeks, Egyptians and Romans, and it was so popular in mediaeval England that a special tax was levied on it! The active ingredient in anise is a volatile oil called anethol which helps your stomach to digest rich foods that you might otherwise struggle to digest. It also helps to settle your stomach and through the stimulation of gastric juice production, it helps to regulate the whole digestion process as well.

CONCLUSION

As you have seen, because irritable bowel syndrome is not a single recognizable illness or disease, there are many different factors and aspects to consider when looking for natural ways of dealing with the problem.

Nevertheless, this does not change the fact that there are many different ways of treating irritable bowel syndrome completely naturally without resorting to chemical-based medical drugs that can have potentially adverse (or possibly even lethal) side-effects, albeit in a very small number of cases.

More importantly, it is crucial to remember that all medical treatments for irritable bowel syndrome are designed to do nothing more than manage the condition.

Most doctors are not going to have the time (or perhaps the inclination) to analyze your condition in enough depth or detail to come up with a sustainable lifestyle-changing plan with which you can attack your IBS problem at a more fundamental level, so in order to do this, it is up to you.

In the majority of cases, medicine treats irritable bowel syndrome on only the most peripheral level, whereas by adopting natural strategies for dealing with the problem, you can quite realistically expect to remove many of the primary causes of IBS attacks from your life.

As you have seen, there is also nothing particularly complicated or complex about making the changes necessary to minimize your susceptibility to irritable bowel syndrome. For example, altering your diet as suggested is something that anyone should be able to do, but this one simple step will make a significant difference to your future susceptibility to IBS problems.

Stress is almost certainly the number one cause of your condition so it is clearly extremely important to deal with stress. In particular, you have to learn to live with it and not allow it to dominate your life. Get on top of your stress, learn how to handle it and remove another significant causative factor from the picture.

The bottom line is, it is not a difficult thing to deal with irritable bowel syndrome naturally.

Everything you need to know is detailed in this manual and now that you are armed with this information, you can start taking appropriate actions immediately.

Printed by Libri Plureos GmbH in Hamburg, Germany